Lavinia

The Little Book of Falling (and Getting Up)

Prevent Injury and Recover Quickly from Gravity's Embrace

Introduction

I've been falling all my life. As a child, I often found myself lying face down in the mud, grass or street without realizing how I got there. One memorable fall pitched me head first down the stairs. Before I could cry, my parents grabbed me, sat me at the kitchen table and served me a bowl of ice cream; a rare treat that perhaps made me forever think that falling down was a good thing.

When I was a young actor, one of my wise teachers told me that we are successful when we turn our liabilities into assets. I became a mime and physical comedienne specializing in dive rolls, prat falls and kicks in the pants. It was nice to get paid for falling down.

But it didn't cure my clumsiness. Offstage I still fell downstairs, on hiking paths, and sidewalks. Sometimes my theater skills helped. Once after a rain, I slipped on some mud while jogging. I tucked, rolled and kept running. A woman came panting up next to me. *"Is that some new kind of aerobic exercise?"* she asked.
Sometimes nothing helped and I had to nurse bruises, sprained ankles and even a couple of bloody noses.

Then I discovered the Feldenkrais Method®. Developed by Dr. Moshe Feldenkrais, the Feldenkrais Method uses small, slow movements combined with awareness that change the way you move, think and act. I had no idea it would affect my falling. I just wanted to stop the aches and pains that seemed to be part of my career. What I discovered was an avenue towards better posture, greater relaxation and more efficient movement. And I learned that while falling is a fact of life, you can develop strategies for both landing more softly as well as swifter recovery.

The exercises in this book are based on Moshe Feldenkrais' teaching. He called his movement sequences Awareness Through Movement® lessons. While it's true that we are often hyper-aware while walking on ice, or crossing a stream, that awareness is often laced with tension.

Awareness Through Movement lessons teach people how to sense their movement, sensations, feelings and thoughts without stress.

We use the word "falling" for countless emotional experiences: falling in love, into debt, out of favor, from grace. Oxford's Dictionary has two pages dedicated to definitions of falling. Over the last twenty years, I've worked with thousands of people. Many had injuries from falling or were afraid of falling. Sometimes it wasn't so much about falling as it was about getting up. Often after studying the movements of the Feldenkrais Method for a while, people come up to me with big grins and said, *"Hey Lavinia, guess what, I fell on the ice yesterday,"* or *"I was working in the garden, pulling weeds and went down!"* These announcements ended with, *"...and amazingly, I didn't hurt a thing!"*

Falling happens so quickly, there's no time for the ordinary thinking brain to make a choice. You have to rely on your kinesthetic intelligence. That's the part of your body/mind that governs your movement habits. Your kinesthetic, or sensory intelligence knows exactly what to do as you back your car out of the driveway, flip an egg or ride your bicycle. While you can't "train yourself to fall", you can develop a more intelligent body that can help you in the event of a fall.

By exploring the movements in this book, you will discover a new way to prepare yourself for the inevitable. All of us are subject to gravity. Why not make it your friend?

How to Use This Book

I've organized this book as a user friendly introduction to aspects of falling and getting up; from the biomechanical to the psychological and metaphoric.
It aims to help you become more flexible and resilient so you are and therefore more able to recover in the event of a fall.

When you get to the exercises, do them slowly, in a relaxed fashion. The motto of the Feldenkrais Method® is "less pain, more gain." Each person does the movements according to his own ability, understanding and interest. If you find something is too difficult to understand or to do, then you are right, your nervous system is not ready.

That doesn't mean you should strain, and it doesn't mean that you won't be able to do it later. Work with the movements that feel pleasurable to do, and eventually, all the movements in this book will be accessible. The sequences in this book are written in a condensed, abbreviated style so you don't have to follow a lot of detail as you move.

However, many people prefer following audio instructions rather than reading them in a book. So I have recorded expanded versions of all these lessons, essentially an entire workshop, which are available for purchase as a CD or MP3 download at www.laviniaplonka.com

There are video clip references for some of the movement lessons, you can find the youtube links at the end of the book. These clips are just for reference, there is no need to imitate them. You have your own way of moving, your own way of responding to instructions. Think of the video as a moving illustration of the instructions in case the words themselves are not enough.

"Fall down eight times, get up nine."
Japanese Proverb

Contents

Fear of Falling/Failing..14

The Gravity of the Situation...23

The Dance Between Stability and Mobility.......................29

Sweet Surrender: The Art of Letting Go............................33

Stepping Up, Over and Around..39

You Make Me Dizzy – That Old Vestibular System
and How to Stay Upright...47

I Get Knocked Down, But I Get Up Again........................53

The Downward (and Upward) Spiral.................................57

Chapter 1
Fear of Falling/Failing

Marjorie came to one of my Falling Workshops. She was an athlete and a trainer with a passion for tennis. Marjorie informed me that she had recently lost her balance on the tennis court and had so severely sprained her ankle that she hadn't been able to return to playing or even to doing all her work. A few months after the workshop, she stopped by the studio. *"I just had to share with you in person,"* she said excitedly, *"that I fell!"*

"Is that a good thing?" I asked.

"Yes!" She exclaimed. *"When I sprained my ankle,"* Marjorie continued, *"I had felt myself losing my balance. But I was so afraid of looking incompetent, or that my students would judge me if I landed on the ground, that I forced myself to stay upright. To onlookers, it merely looked like I stumbled a bit, but in the process I made my injury worse. Then I jogged off the court trying to look good, doing even more damage. This time, as I ran up to the net, my shoe got caught and I went off balance. Instead of trying to "hold it together," I let the racket fly from my hand, softened my knees and rolled in the dirt. I was immediately surrounded by a dozen worried people.*

Are you OK?' they all asked.

I rolled to my side, and spiraled up to standing, shook myself off, and thought about it. 'Yes, I'm totally fine,' I replied. And I was! I didn't worry about looking ridiculous and I had landed softly and injury free."

There are three main reasons to fear falling. The first two:

fear of injury, and the fear that you will be unable to get up, are physiological fears based in our instinct for self-preservation. Falling is like diving into the unknown: you can't predict the outcome, which is scary enough. Who needs a cut lip, a broken arm or hip? Add the specter of brittle bones and this possibility becomes more threatening. And if you don't think you can get back up after landing, the idea of falling makes you more nervous.

The third reason people fear falling is psychological: a fear of "looking stupid." Like Marjorie, many people feel that falling is a humiliation. The inability to stay upright implies some failure, like falling down on the job.

> *What would life be if we had no courage*
> *to attempt anything?*

> Vincent van Gogh

Studies show that fear of falling actually increases the chances of falling. If you are afraid, you are tense. Being tense while walking limits your vision, range of motion, and ability to recover balance in a dangerous situation. There is hesitancy, tension, inability to focus on what's necessary. Failure, like falling, is like a date with destiny. It's a learning experience that's bound to happen at some time. Marjorie's connection between fear of falling and failing was literal. Some people so utterly fear failure, they never even attempt the dream they have in their hearts.

We have many sayings relating success/failure to falling. "He fell flat on his face." "She landed on her feet." "The higher you climb, the harder you fall." When we fall in public, we remind everyone of our vulnerability. You failed to "stay on your feet." Slapstick comedy capitalizes on this. Everyone laughs at the clown who slips on the banana peel. So even if the fall is painful, and no one around you is laughing, you feel as silly as the clown who just catapulted into a vegetable bin or mud puddle. It implies you made a wrong move. You weren't paying attention. You are obviously, in front of the entire world, less than perfect. That fear of embarrassment can paralyze you. In some cultures, even up till modern times, embarrassment, or "losing face" could even lead to suicide.

Can developing physical skills that improve balance and flexibility help people "take the plunge" metaphorically as well: in a new relationship, career move, or venture? Science has not yet figured out an effective measurement for something like this. However, common sense can tell you that if you are relaxed, you are more balanced, more ready to respond to whatever situations may arise.

Feldenkrais often said, "It's not flexible bodies I'm after, it's flexible brains." He was one of the first people to state that there is not just a mind/body connection, but that the mind and the body are one and the same. To call it a connection would be like saying the mind lives in one part and the body lives someplace else, communicating by some corporeal telephone. If the body is better organized, then the mind also functions better. If you know you have strategies for recovery, you won't be paralyzed by fear.

Lesson #1
Falling from the Floor

In order to overcome the fear of falling, it's best to begin close to the ground. That way you don't have far to go and can easily recognize when fear inhibits movement. I often work privately with people who have a lot of pain. We work on a low table, where I use gentle movement to help them discover new options for better function. Sometimes students while lying on their side, are very stiff, as if holding themselves in place. As I encourage a little rolling action to the back, they will suddenly pull back to the original position. When I ask them what happened, they often say, *"I was about to fall!"*

"You felt you were going to fall off the table?" I ask.
"Noooo," you can already hear the shock. *"I was afraid I would fall from my side onto my back...onto the table...."*
At which point, they usually start laughing.

So before we begin to learn "how to fall" we want to address the fear in a safe environment, by practicing the feeling of falling "from the floor."
You will need some space for this exercise, at least an arm's width to each side of yourself while lying on your back. If you can't find a floor space like this in your home or office, or if you have difficulty getting to the floor, you can do it lying crossways across your bed.

Bend your knees and bring them up over your chest. Hold your right knee with your right hand, your left knee with your left hand. Begin to gently rock left and right.

Notice how you do this movement. Do both of your legs go together, or does one lead? What does your head do? As you roll, do you inhale, exhale, or hold your breath? What do you feel in your head? In your neck?

Let go of your legs and take a rest. Give yourself a moment to check in.
How do you feel? Relaxed? Stressed? Tired? All of this is information. If you feel stressed or tired, give yourself permission to rest longer, or even give it up for today, returning to it later to try again.

Take the same position as before. This time, as you begin the movement, can you let one of your legs lead to the side? When you roll to your right, let your right leg separate from your left leg, and then the left leg follows, and vice versa.
Now what happens? What do you feel happening between your legs? Are you rolling more or rolling less? Pay attention to your head. Is it rolling or staying still?
For a few movements, keep your head still. How far can you roll while holding your head in place?

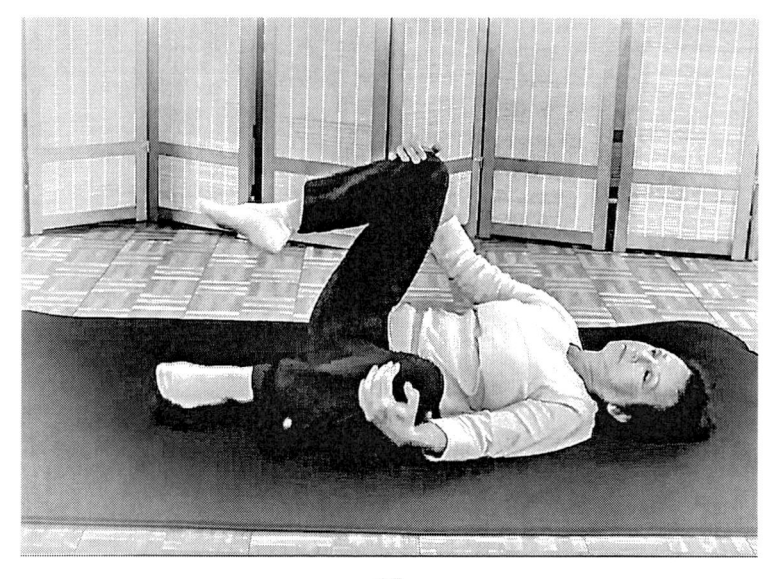

Now roll your head along with your leading leg. Can you roll further? Can you roll all the way to one side? How does that feel? And now what are you going to do? How do you roll back to your back? How do you roll to the other side? Or are you stuck?

Many people get stuck on the side, feeling that their only option is to hurl themselves up and over.
From lying on your side try this: Lift your top leg only. Start going over towards the other side. Before you move your lower leg, allow your pelvis to roll. Roll your head along with your leg. Your other leg comes up last, after everything else has rolled as far as you can go.

Rest again.

A Note on Resting
Every exercise in this book contains many rests.

Pausing after doing some movement gives your body a chance to digest and integrate what you just experienced. It may seem like you are doing very little, yet by taking your time, paying attention and resting, you will improve much more rapidly than by rushing and forcing. So take the invitation to rest seriously.

Notice if this sequence has been fun, scary, painful, or interesting. Maybe you have some other adjective to describe it. If you felt anxiety, fear or tension as you did this, try the exercise again at another time, giving yourself permission to stop whenever you choose. Feel free to go on to the other exercises in the book. In fact, doing other lessons and then returning to the beginning is a great way to increase your learning.

**Gravity.
It isn't just a good idea.
It's the law.**

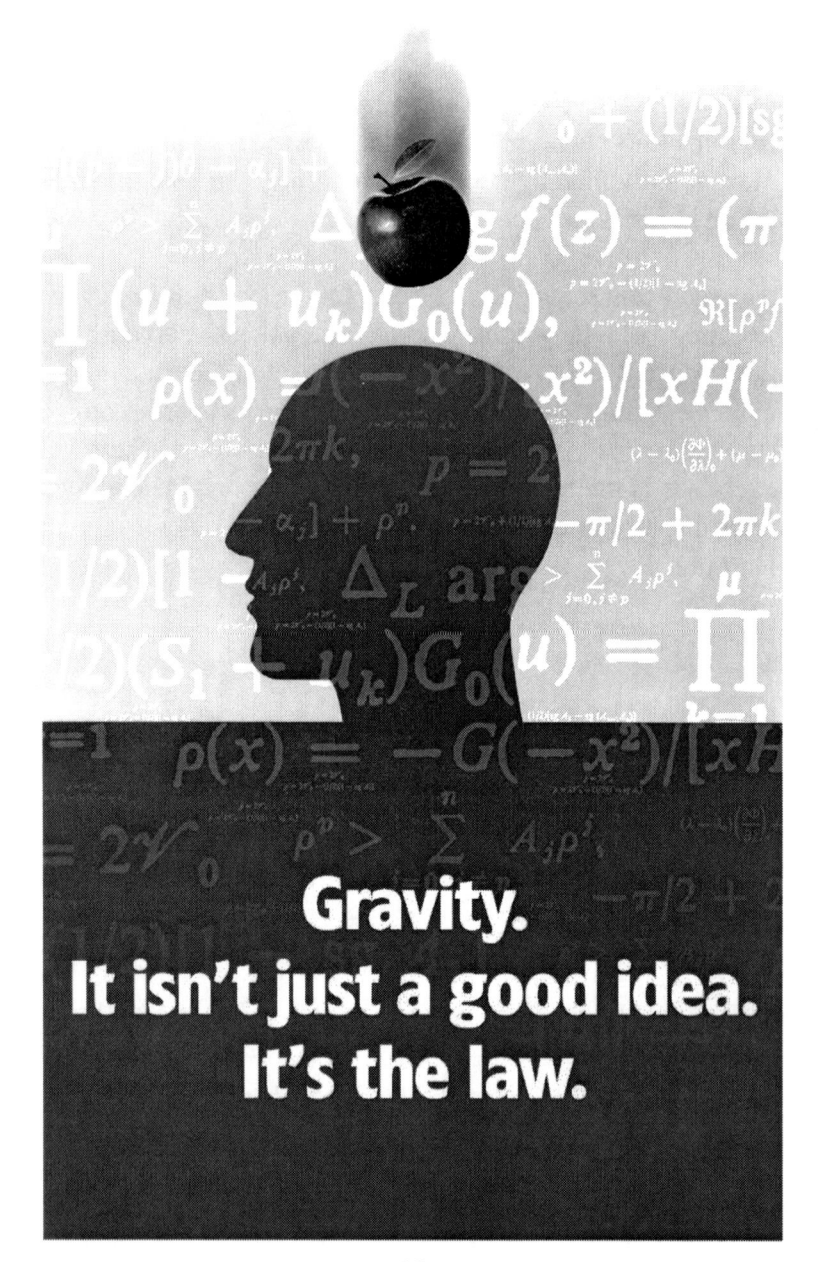

Chapter 2
The Gravity of the Situation

Every time we get up to walk, reach to the top shelf for a dish, or lift an object, no matter how light, we are reckoning with gravity, which is everywhere. Like asking a fish, "How's the water?" we can't describe our relationship to gravity.

Humans live in a very precarious relationship with this force. Unlike four legged creatures whose weight is distributed in a very stable fashion, we have between five and seven feet of skeleton, muscle and flesh perched on two tiny supports: our feet.

Recently Daniel Lieberman, an evolutionary biologist at Harvard, stated that humans were designed for running[2]. Not standing still, but moving rapidly through space. So when there is a crack in the sidewalk, a surprise change in level (Watch Your Step!), or the proverbial roller skate in the hallway, motion is interrupted. Gravity wins and we fall down.

An interruption of forward momentum is a shock to the body. When we experience shock; whether it's a loud noise or a sudden loss of balance, we tend to react in what is called the startle reflex. The body spontaneously first arches and tenses, and then if there's time, curls into a ball.

Some biologists have theorized that this instinctive reaction is left over from our arboreal ancestors falling out of trees. After the shock of missing a branch, the animal could curl up and roll. But a fall from walking is too fast. We arch the back and tense (1) hitting the ground hard before curling up (2) can protect us.

(1)   (2)

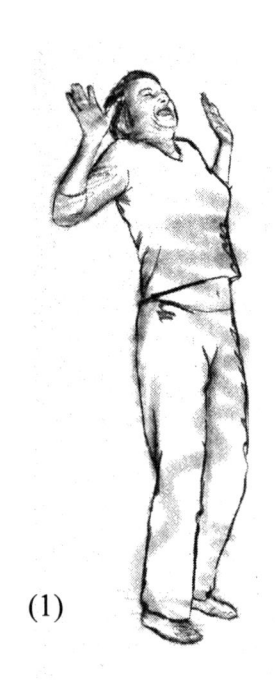

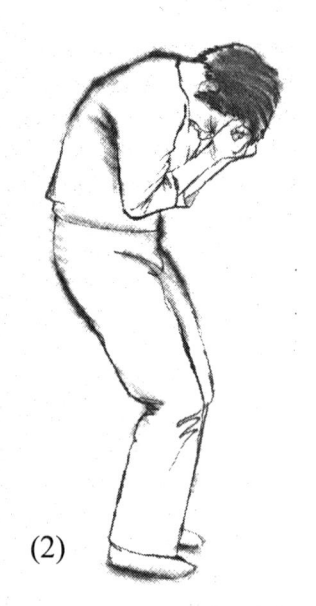

© Ron Morecraft

Learning to "roll with it" is an important strategy when you fall, but also in life. It's easy to get stuck in the startle response: when the boss calls, an unexpected bill arrives in the mail or some other "situation of immense gravity" pulls you out of your comfort zone, making you tense up and limiting your options. By developing physical resilience, you'll discover you have emotional flexibility as well.

When Mark's father died, he assumed he would share an inheritance. He was devastated to find that his siblings were trying to cut him out. He became defensive and angry, adding fuel to the fire. His back went into spasm and he couldn't even walk. He came to see me for the pain. One day, as he allowed his back to soften so he could roll, he had an "aha!"

moment. He recognized a series of fears – everything from fear of being cheated to fear of being an imposter. All of it was held in his breath and his back. His back pain disappeared as he said, "It's only money, why am I killing myself?" Shortly after that he and his siblings amicably settled the estate.

While not every grave situation affects the back, there's no better way to free yourself from the effects of gravity, either physical or emotional, then learning how to roll. It not only softens the spine, it allows you to literally see the world from another angle. Developing the ability to roll can help you in the event of any interruption of your momentum: physical, professional or in relationships. There are many ways to explore rolling. Here is one that explores not just gravity, but how you can use momentum to bring yourself back up.

Lesson #2
Returning From the Point of No Return

Lie down on the floor or your bed and check that you have at least eight inches above your head. After you have made sure you have room above your head when lying down for this exercise, sit back up.

Stretch out your legs on the floor and interlace your fingers behind your right knee. Lower your head towards your knee as if you wanted to rest your forehead on your thigh, don't try to touch. Your elbows will bend. Keeping your head bent and back rounded, slowly go backwards as if you were going to lie down, letting your arms get long, then bend your arms again and return to being bent over your leg. Don't let go of your leg and make sure your arms straighten as you move away, then bend as you return. Try this a few times till it feels easy.

Continue moving backwards, your right knee will bend up, dragging your foot towards you. Don't lift your foot off the floor. (That's the point of no return!) You'll find you are rolling backwards a bit. Keep your arms straight.

Come back up, straightening your right leg so it pulls your arms and you sit with your head lowered toward your thigh. Repeat this a few times till it feels easy.

Rest. Repeat the entire above sequence using your left leg, then rest.

When you sit up again, start with the same movement, but keep rolling backwards. This time your foot eventually comes off the floor. You will end up rolling on your back. As you "fall" backwards keep looking at your thigh, in other words, keep your back rounded. If you let your head fall backwards, your back will straighten out and you will be stuck when you land. If you keep round, it will be easy to just stretch out your right leg to roll right back up! If you find you land and can't get back up without force, rest, come up to sitting in the easiest way possible, and try again.

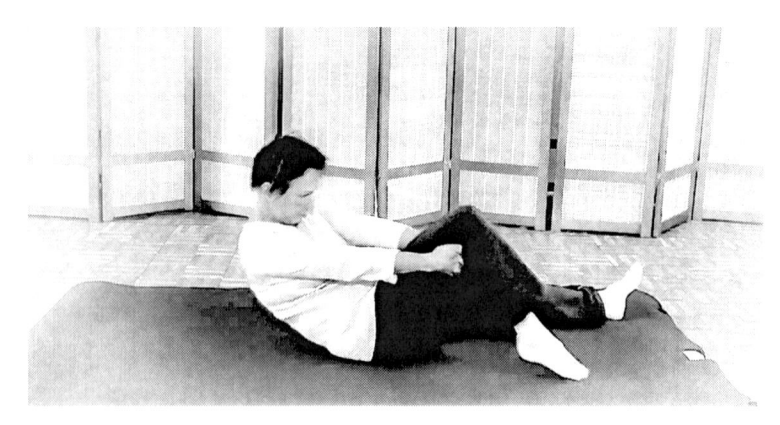

Don't try to "muscle" your way back up.

"Insanity: doing the same thing over and over again and expecting different results."
Albert Einstein

After doing it a few times, regardless of how far you get, take a rest. Then try it with your left leg.

Three important clues:

1) When you roll backwards, let your body pull your leg. Keep your arms straight till you are on your back. To return, let your leg pull your arms so that the arms straighten.

2) Breathe! If you hold your breath, your arms and shoulders will tense. By practicing an easy breath in this approximation of falling, your body will learn to stay more relaxed in the event of a real fall.

3) And remember, it's not important to get back up. What is important is to pay attention to how you are feeling as you explore the movement. If you feel tense, judgmental or frustrated, chances are you do that in your life as well.

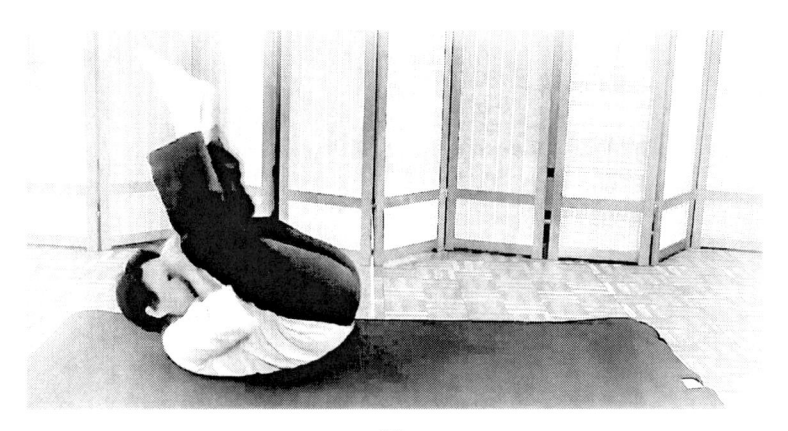

Chapter 3
The Dance Between Stability and Mobility

Picture a tango. The dancers execute a series of steps across the floor, suddenly stop, turn their heads or pose, then quickly change direction to sweep across the floor. It's thrilling to watch a good dance team as they shift from stillness to movement. Most of us wouldn't think of our own life as a dance, and yet it is. Consider making breakfast. You walk into the kitchen, then stop exactly by the coffee pot. Without a second thought, you turn to the sink and fill the pot with water, executing another smooth turn back to the coffeemaker. A few perfectly timed steps bring you to the cabinet or refrigerator, another stop to grab the coffee. Every part of the breakfast choreography is filled with movement and pauses, all perfectly timed to end with your seated position at the table. I can almost hear the music.

But what happens when the dance is interrupted? The cat running under your feet. Dropping the cereal box. The phone ringing just as you're pouring the coffee. In the theater, this would be a call to improvise. Actors are trained to "think on their feet" and look for options that can save the scene. But often we are thrown off balance, literally, simply because we don't know how to recover without freezing, or we are too stuck in wanting to be stable.

Lesson #3
Softening the Ankles

Here are a few experiments to help you explore stability and mobility. Stand perfectly still. If you can stand with your eyes closed, great, but this can work with your eyes open as well. Notice your ankles.

Are they tense? Many people can't tell what's going on down there. If you're not sure, tighten your ankles for two breaths and then let go. Do they feel different?

You will begin to sway. As the swaying increases, some of you may even notice that the swaying begins to take on a figure eight pattern. Our ankles are an important part of our circulatory system. The movement of blood makes us want to move. Now tighten your ankles so that you don't sway, and notice what happens then.

Some people start to feel tension in other parts. Others stop breathing. When you tense your ankles, you affect your circulation. Poor circulation has been shown to create balance problems, as does holding your breath.

Stand with your feet parallel. Let your body rock forward. What happens? Eventually you will fall forward and have to catch yourself. Rock backwards on your heels. Yikes! Who would think our habitual way of standing is so unstable? No wonder our ankles get tense.

Place one foot a little bit in front of the other, as if you just took a step. Rock forward so the weight goes on your front foot. Does that feel more stable? The most that happens is you end up taking a step forward. Same thing if you step backwards.

Tightening up or suddenly stopping are two easy ways to fall down. And yet, our fear/startle reactions cause us to do exactly that. If instead of trying to stop the fall, you keep your feet going, you will defuse the impact and have more options for recovering your balance. If you are in movement, it's much easier to land gracefully, making even a fall look like part of a dance.

Shirley is "on the other side of 80" as she puts it. While visiting New York City, she accidentally stepped off a curb and lost her balance, falling onto the sidewalk. She said it felt like she was descending in slow motion as she watched herself roll onto the sidewalk. Because she's such a frail looking elder, she was immediately surrounded by people who wanted to help. One man commented as he brushed off her dress. "*Wow. That was the most graceful fall I've ever seen.*" Outside of a bruise on her hip, Shirley was uninjured. She credits her Feldenkrais classes.

Doing the above ankle exercises can help you improve your chances of interrupting a fall, or falling gracefully.

Chapter 4
Sweet Surrender or the Art of Letting Go

There are entire books written about how to let go. There are over twenty published poems titled "Let Go and Let God." We're encouraged to let go of our baggage, our story, our past, our fear.

We can draw a connection between the gripping that takes place when we try not to fall and the rigidity of trying to hold on to the past, security, old story, or whatever else keeps us from surrendering. Western culture generally disapproves of surrender, as if it implies a disgraceful defeat. Yet we surrender every day. When we yield in traffic, hand over money to a cashier, acknowledge that someone was right, or open the door for someone, we are surrendering.

When I work one on one with people, I have the pleasure of guiding their attention while moving and lifting different parts of their bodies, allowing them to learn to let go of habitual holdings that steal energy, create muscular tension and pain, and lead to problems ranging from headaches to arthritis. Often when I lift a leg or an arm, people are shocked to discover that they cannot let go or give me their weight. Their need to hold on and control comes in direct conflict with the invitation to surrender to someone else's support. More than once, I've raised someone's arm and felt them trying to control the movement, even with their eyes closed. "*Just let go,*" I'll say.

"*I am letting go,*" is often the reply. So I will release the arm (in a safe position) and the arm just hangs in the air. Even then, the person will sometimes insist that the arm is completely relaxed, hanging up in the air, although more often, they are simply shocked.

When you learn how to "let go" in a fall, you are less prone to injury than if you grip and resist. I have found that people who are having difficulty letting go; of a relationship, a habit, or a fear, are able to use Feldenkrais lessons to relieve the emotional tension associated with "holding on." When the body is more relaxed, it's a lot easier to see the way more clearly. Tension literally affects vision. So if you can't see the world clearly, you can't see your life situations clearly either.

"Find your true weakness and surrender to it. Therein lies the path to genius. Most people spend their lives using their strengths to overcome or cover up their weaknesses. Those few who use their strengths to incorporate their weaknesses, who don't divide themselves, those people are very rare."
Moshe Feldenkrais

Lesson #4
Surrendering Your Body Parts

This lesson will have more impact (literally) if you can do it lying on a mat on the floor. But if you feel unsafe, or it's too difficult to get down to the floor, then stick with the bed.

Many people fear breaking bones when they fall, having an image of the bones as stiff, brittle sticks. But your bones are so much more than that. They are living tissue. The marrow of our bones is literally where our blood supply is made. The bones are designed to be strong and vital.

Because of their structure, a solid exterior and soft interior, our bones also resonate and vibrate; helping us sense the ground and our distance from walls and objects. If we stiffen as we fall, we don't allow the joints to relax. The bones can't adjust where they will land, therefore injury occurs. In this lesson, we'll explore how dropping your bones can help you surrender to gravity without stiffness or injury.

Lie on your back with your arms comfortably by your side. If it's easy, leave your legs stretched out. But if your back feels uncomfortable, for now, bend your knees and put your feet flat on the floor. Pick up your right arm a couple of inches off the floor and drop it. Don't lift it high, and don't control the descent. Just let it fall to the ground. Of course, the higher you lift, the harder the crash, the more anxiety you may provoke. So stay within your comfort range and pay attention to your breath. Raise and drop your arm several times. Rest.

Try the same thing with your left arm. Rest.

Return to lifting and dropping your right arm, but this time, when it's up in the air, turn it over. One time you land on the palm side, one time on the back side of the hand. If it feels easy, speed it up. See if you can still yield and land with a "thunk" when you speed up. If you find yourself tensing up, or holding back from surrender, don't lift so high. Rest. Do the same thing with the left arm.

When we fall, it's fast. Learning to let go lightly and quickly will help your nervous system rapidly respond in the event of a real fall. This principle of learning to let your body parts go is crucial to landing softly. If you can't surrender while you're lying on the floor, it will be even harder to let go while falling.

Try the same thing with your legs. To do this you need to

stretch your legs out. First try just lifting and dropping one leg. Then add turning your leg in the air before it lands. It doesn't have to be a lot.

What happens as you speed up? Do you tense up? Maybe the leg stays loose but the rest of you is holding on. Pay attention. Notice how you resist surrender. Notice as your body parts land, how you feel the vibration through the rest of your body. That means your bones are conducting force. Have you ever wondered why martial artists slap the floor when they fall? It's to absorb the shock through their bones. What other body parts can you throw into the air? Your shoulders? Your head? Lift your pelvis a bit and let it drop. Combine body parts. An arm and a leg. The head and the arms. Allow yourself to play.

Chapter 5
Stepping Up, Over and Around

Long ago, people rode in horse-drawn carriages on bumpy dirt roads through forests and fields. The carriage axles were designed to lubricate themselves as they hit bumps, releasing grease that kept the machinery running smoothly. As cities developed smoother roads, these carriages no longer experienced these "shocks" to their structure, so the greasing action didn't happen. This was fine, until the carriage hit a bump, when the whole mechanism often fell apart because the axle had rusted.

Humans are designed in a similar fashion. Our joints are lubricated by synovial fluid that keeps them flexible and supple. When we engage in varied activities, or travel on uneven terrain, the joints maintain their lubrication. However if we always walk on paved roads, treadmills or in malls, the hips, like the carriage, will not be prepared for the challenges of a sudden change in surface – whether it's a crack in the sidewalk, an unexpected ledge or a pothole.

People often sense this vulnerability and end up looking down as they walk, further compromising their stability. Your head weighs between eight and twelve pounds. If it's bent forward, you are already heading down towards the ground, plus you can't see what's ahead or around you (we'll look at that more in the next chapter).

One of the best ways to lubricate your joints is to go hiking on a mountain trail. The rocks, twists and turns, and changes in level can make your hip joints very happy, even if you go slowly and not very far. But not everyone has a mountain in their back yards, so we need some simple movements that can offer similar benefits. The hip joints are located inside your pelvis and need the action of the pelvis to move efficiently. When you step over a rock, duck under a bush, squeeze around a puddle, you are using your pelvis in concert with your hips. When walking on a straight road, it's easy to forget how the pelvis supports movement. Many people just move the legs, effectively freezing parts of the body. If you learn to include your pelvis in your image of walking, you will fall far less often and will save your hips from potential wear and tear.

I invited the class to walk around the room and observe how they walk. *"What is your pelvis doing?"* I asked.
"My pelvis?" an older man laughed. *"I haven't thought about my pelvis in years!"*

After working with a woman who had severe hip and knee pain for several sessions, she got up from a lesson and began to walk. Her hips swayed elegantly and her walk, which had been stiff and ungainly, was now smooth. She stopped in the middle of the room. *"Oh my,"* she exclaimed. *"I'm walking like a hussy!"*

Our culture has emphasized the sexual aspect of pelvic movement and forgotten the functional. Reclaiming the mobility and power of the pelvis is a study unto itself. For our purposes, I ask only that you suspend your previous conceptions of "proper walking" and enjoy the following exploration.

The Planes of Pelvic Motion
The pelvis has three ways that it can move: forward and back, twisting (rotating) right and left, and side bending (one hip going up to the shoulder, bending the ribs).

There are many ways to explore the way the pelvis is involved in walking. The following lesson is done standing, so we can experience the movement in our verticality.

Lesson #5
Forward and Back

Take a chair and stand behind it so that you can rest your hands on the back of the chair. Alternatively, you can stand near a wall where you can put your hands on the wall for balance. Begin by repeating the movement you did in Chapter 3, swaying forward and back. Now shift your weight to the right leg, and then the left leg.

Notice how you shift your weight. What does your pelvis do to make that happen?

Begin to raise and lower your right heel. As you raise your heel, bend your right knee. Place your right hand on your hip bone (the big bone on the top right part of your pelvis) as you raise and lower your heel.

Does it move? What do you feel happening there?

Your pelvis can tilt slightly as your heel comes up. Your back rounds a little bit, your tailbone tucking under slightly. Everything straightens as your heel comes down. As you raise and lower your heel, you create a slight rocking motion. Do it slowly, and then more quickly. To rest, sit down in your chair, or take a walk around.
Try the same movement with the left heel. Does this side move differently? Rest.

Come back to standing behind your chair. This time, begin to pick up the front of your right foot, rocking back on the heel. Feel how your pelvis can tilt so that your back arches slightly and your tailbone reaches backward. Try going both ways, once lifting your heel, once lifting the ball of your foot. Rest, then try it on the left.

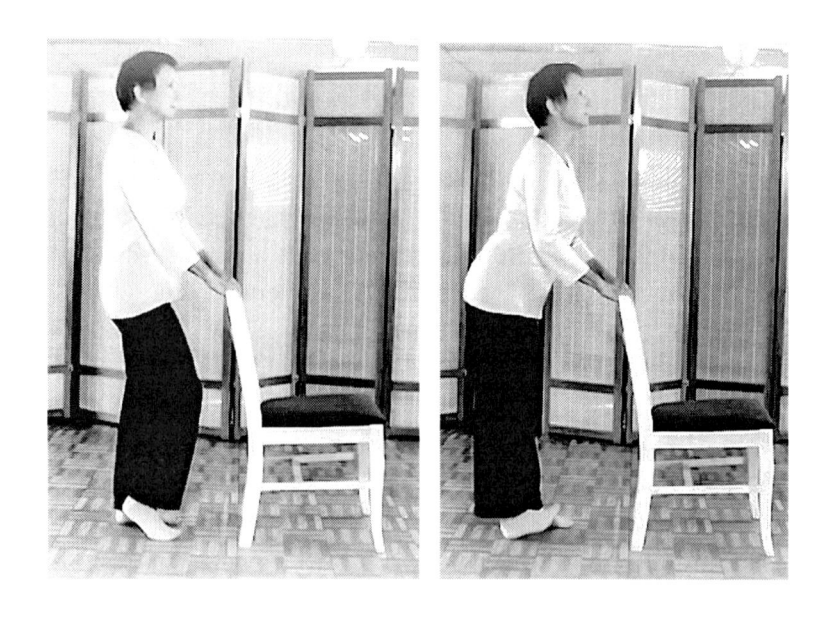

If you feel secure, you can explore this further by rocking on both feet at the same time. If you do this, don't push to the extreme, keep it small but interesting.

One of the mottos of the Feldenkrais Method is "Less is more." By keeping the movement small and simple, you have more mental space to pay attention to how you do the movement. Take another rest.

Rotation
Resume your position behind the chair. Pick up your right heel and swivel it out to the right, then place it on the floor. Your right foot will look pigeon toed. Bring it back to center. Then pick up the right heel and swivel it left, putting it down so that your foot is now turned out. Bring it back to center. Begin to alternate where you place your heel. Swivel once to the right, stand on it, come to the center, stand on it, left, stand on it, and return to the center. Once you get this movement going, can you notice what's happening to your

pelvis? You may feel it's turning a little. Go ahead and let that happen. As your heel swivels right, let your pelvis turn a bit to the left. As your heel swivels left, turn your pelvis to the right. Take a rest, then try it with your left foot. If you feel like doing both heels, move them together. You may start to feel like a skier!

Side Bending
Stand with your feet comfortably apart. Begin sliding your right hand down the side of your leg towards your knee and come back up.

As you slide your arm down, notice what your ribs want to do. Can you feel how the ribs on your left expand while the ribs on the right come together? What happens to your weight? Does it shift to the right or the left?

Play with shifting your weight to one foot or the other as you reach down. Rest. Do the same thing on the left side. When you get to the part where you shift your weight, try lifting a

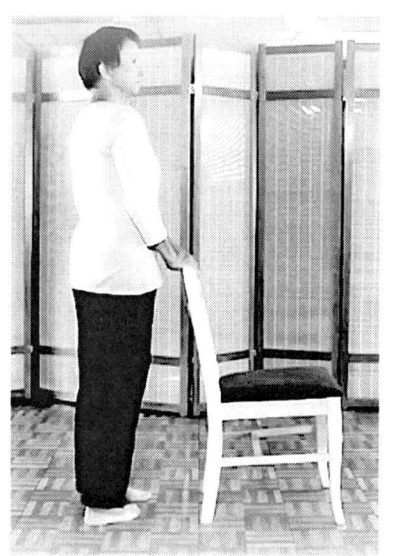

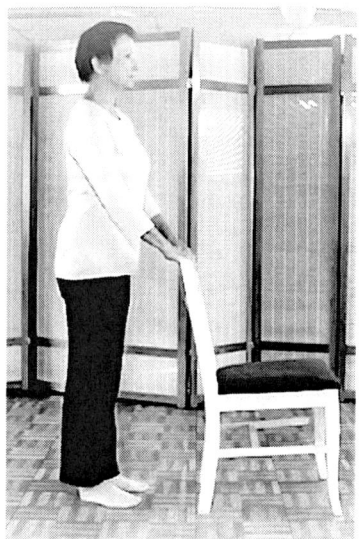

heel. If this feels unstable, place your non-reaching hand on the back of your chair, and do one side at a time.
Which heel feels good to lift? Which one lets your arm go down more easily? Do your hips move? Which way?
Rest.

Take a fresh stance and simply shift your weight right and left. What does it feel like now?

Then take a walk, even if it's just from one room to the other. What attracts your attention? Your feet? Your weight? Your posture? Each time you do these movements, you may discover something new about yourself.

Chapter 6
You Make Me Dizzy: That Old Vestibular System, and How to Stay Upright

When I was a child, I liked to twirl and twirl as fast as I could, and then stop. For a few delicious minutes, the world kept spinning around me. Sometimes it was so intense, I fell over. When we are young, falling down can actually be fun. Of course, children are much closer the ground, their bones are less brittle, their muscles softer. Nowadays, if the world starts spinning, we often reach for the nearest chair to avoid falling down.

As I mentioned before, four legged creatures have little fear of falling. But being bipedal, besides making us unstable, also gives us advantages. We have the ability to use the hands for other tasks. And we can rotate and look around, even while walking. That allows us to take in more of the environment.

The human vestibular system is a whole body experience. In my fabulous experience of twirling, that crazy feeling of the world spinning around was the result of the fluid in my ear canal. When you spin, it's sloshing back and forth in your head. When you stop, it takes a few moments to settle, giving you that unsettling feeling that the world is moving without you.

People who suffer from various forms of vertigo find this less than pleasant. Anyone who has had an ear infection that affected balance, or who suffers from vertigo, has experienced a challenge with this aspect of the vestibular system.

Another key component of the vestibular system is your

skeleton. Remember in Chapter 4 when you threw your body parts into the air and dropped them? Each time your bones touch something, you are sending information to your vestibular system: your feet hitting the floor with each step, your hand reaching out to grab a doorknob, your nose when you bump into the bathroom wall in the middle of the night. Your bones conduct vibrations that carry on a lively dialogue with that ear canal.

Your eyes do more than see, they are also an integral part of the vestibular system, helping you orient in space. Several sets of muscles, as well as the lenses in your eyes (not your contact lenses, but your actual eye) are constantly adjusting to objects near and far, and the environment that surrounds you, including what is above and below. The brain processes all this information to keep you upright. As your eyes move, the movement engages muscles in the neck, back, jaw and even the feet.

Refer back to Lesson #3 where you explored standing still with eyes open and closed. If you try the exercise again with your eyes closed and then open, you will see that it's much more difficult to stay upright with your eyes closed.

Interestingly, people who have tension in their eyes also suffer from balance problems. If the eyes have gotten into a habit of just looking forward, perhaps from sitting at a computer or a lot of driving, this can often create a lot of tension in the neck and shoulders. This limits options in a moment of instability like when you trip, or someone bumps into you.

By relaxing the eyes, you will find you feel more stable and more flexible at the same time.
The message you send to your vestibular system is "all is good, I'm upright and comfortable."

Lesson #6
Eyes in the Back of Your Head

Stand with your feet comfortably underneath you. Extend your right arm directly in front of you. Pretend that your nose is connected to your right hand with a string so that wherever your arm goes, your head follows.

Begin to turn to the right, everything turning together, your arm, head and trunk. Your eyes are always looking at your hand, not going past the hand, and not letting the hand move from the center of your vision. Turn only as far as is easy and comfortable while keeping everything connected.

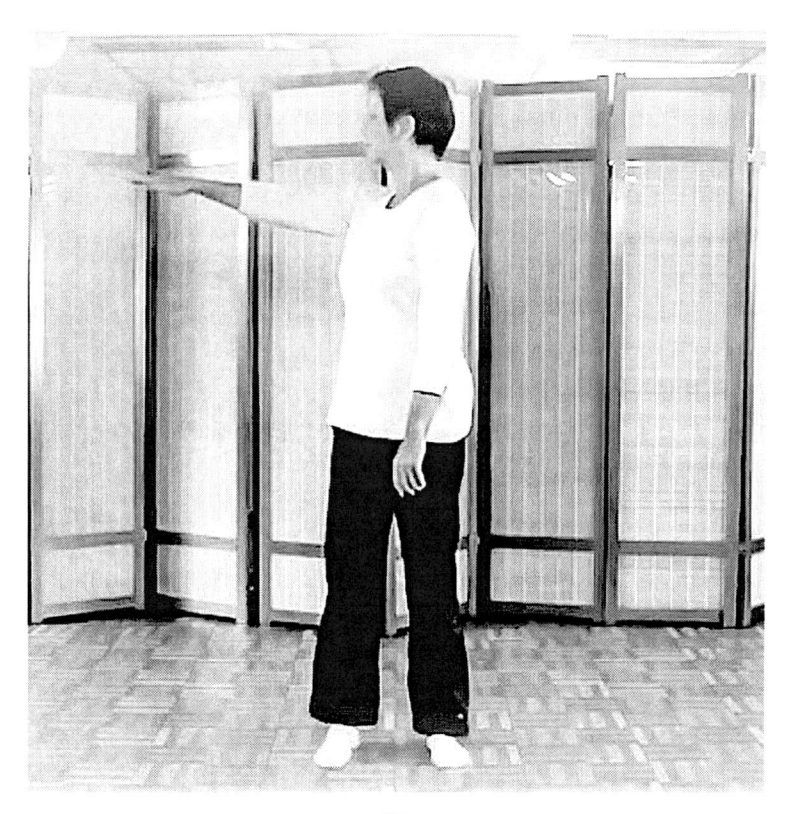

Keep your feet stable.

After a few turns, stay turned to your right.
If your arm is tired you can put it down, but keep your face and trunk turned to the right. Without moving your trunk, slowly turn your head left and right. Don't strain, and don't go to your limit. What's important is that you pay attention to how you turn, not how far.

After turning your head five or ten times, return everything to face the front. Raise your right arm in front of you again if you had put it down. Turn everything again to the right.
 How are you turning? What are you sensing? How much of the room can you see now?

Take a rest. You can sit down in a chair, lie down or just take a stroll around. After resting, return to the same spot, facing the same way in the room. Raise your right arm again. Turn to your right again and stay there. This time, move only your eyes left and right. This is not always as easy as it sounds, so be kind to yourself.

Take it slowly. Notice how your eyes travel. Do they go in a line? An arc? Smooth? Jumpy? Do they like to go more in one direction than another? Can you keep your head still or does it want to join in?

Return to the front and then see what it's like to turn to your right again.

If you feel like taking things even further, you can do another sequence like this where your eyes look in one direction while your head turns in the other direction.

It's really fun if you're not attached to "getting it right!" Take a walk around and notice what your peripheral vision feels like, your sense of stability, your ability to turn. Is it different from right to left? Try the whole sequence to the other side.

Chapter 7
I Get Knocked Down, But I Get Up Again

*"Each time I find myself lying flat on my face,
I pick myself up and get back in the race."*
　　　　　　　　　　　　　　Frank Sinatra

Next to victory, humans love to celebrate recovery. Whether it's from abuse, alcoholism, bankruptcy, or a KO punch in the ring, there is inner cheering whenever we see someone "…pick myself up, dust myself off and start all over again." Not having the option to get back up is the ultimate defeat. Life Alert made a fortune from a commercial years ago portraying various seniors lying on the ground and calling the service saying, "Help! I've fallen and I can't get up!" The idea that I can't get back up is a harbinger for each of us of the day that we indeed will not get up at the end of our lives.

While it's true that some people's illnesses or injuries prevent them from being able to get down or up from the floor, many more can improve their chances by understanding the principles involved in getting up. Paradoxically, once you learn how to get up from a fall, you will learn to fall "better".

Defeat or collapse implies that you've run out of options. But another way to look at it is: there's no way to go but up! Here's where we once again encounter our friend, gravity. If you try to just pop back up (unless you are eight years old or in Cirq Du Soleil), you encounter resistance. Sometimes the shortest distance between two points is not a straight line, but a spiral.

Lesson #7
Get On Up

As mentioned earlier, a common fear is not being able to get back up from a fall. There are times of course, when a fall leads to a severe injury, a broken bone for example. Those times it's often better to wait for help. Certainly if you fear a severe injury, it's wise to invest in some kind of medical alert service.

Many times there is little to no injury. But stiffness and fragility make getting back up seem impossible. That's where you need to begin to access the intelligence of the skeleton's design as a lever to lift you up. Most people try to haul themselves up, using their backs and arm muscles. Their legs are weak and can't support the lifting of the trunk.

In order to figure out how to get up, we first want to find a safe way to get down. If you have knee problems, take a moment to put some extra padding down on the floor in front of your chair. While we won't be putting much weight on the knee, you always put your comfort first.

Sit on the edge of your chair with your feet flat. Begin swiveling your knees left and right. As you swivel from side to side, notice what you feel in your buttocks underneath you. Does the weight shift at all? Now continue swiveling just to your right a few times. Place your right hand somewhere behind you on the seat of your chair for support.

Both knees move to the right. As you swivel to the right, notice how your left knee drops down a little bit. Go ahead and let that happen. You swivel to the right, and your left knee starts lowering to the floor. You'll feel your left buttock sliding off the chair. Of it feels secure, continue until you feel you can place your left knee on the floor. You are now kneeling and facing the right with your right hand on the chair seat. Now how do you get back in the chair?

Here you discover a paradox. Instead of trying to use your leg muscles to push yourself up, you will go down to get up. Bend your body forward so that your left hand is on the floor somewhere near your right foot. Lower your head as if you want to kiss your knee.

Give a little press with your left hand and raise your buttocks up, then slide them back onto your seat. Don't lift your head till you're in contact with the chair. Remember, it's heavy. If you look up while you're trying to get into the chair, you strain your back. Instead, you want to think of your spine as a lever with the pelvis on one end and the head on the other. Try the movement a few times, each time making it easier. Don't rush, and don't feel you have to get there today.

If coming down to the floor feels too difficult for you, just do the first part of the movement and imagine the rest as you listen to the instructions. Or you can swivel your knees and feet to the right on your chair, lower your head, press your right hand down and just stand up. Keep your head down till your legs are stable. Bring your pelvis forward and your head comes up!

Take a rest, then try the same movement to the left.

Our culture seems to associate dignity with "keeping your head up," as if in some way that implies that you haven't lost your balance. But that only works when you are up on your two feet. If you're down on the ground, using your limbs as a tripod and lifting your true center of gravity is actually much more graceful than muscling yourself up.

Chapter 8
The Shortest Distance
Isn't Always a Straight Line

Most people fall hard because they go straight down, either throwing their hands out, or crashing onto their sides. And when coming from lying or sitting, the tendency is to try to get straight up, as if moving in a straight line will get them there faster.

But there is a more efficient way to come up, and by learning this, you may also discover more options for both balance and recovery when you trip. Instead of crashing straight down, or muscling back up, you can use nature's power of the spiral. Spiraling is actually one of the most efficient ways to get down to the ground and get back up.

As you noticed in the last exercise, you swiveled to your seat, you didn't just pop up. The spiral design is intrinsic in our universe: from the design of our galaxy, to the wind up of a discus thrower, from the inside of a nautilus shell to the seedpods of certain flowers.

The spiral allows us to move in concert with wind resistance, gravity, and perhaps other forces we don't even see. Seedlings emerge by spiraling outward. Watch a figure skater spiral down and up.

Learning how to embody spiraling can soften your landing, and most importantly, help you get back up. While it's true that in most falling scenarios you can't control your descent, developing the flexibility to turn around yourself can often help prevent more serious injuries.

Lesson #8
Upward and Downward Spiral

If you did not manage to get down to the floor in the last chapter, put a second chair in front of where you are sitting. You will be doing an approximation of the spiral. Alternatively, you can have someone help you down to sit on the floor so you can do as much of the movement as feels comfortable. Always consider your comfort and safety first. You can always sit quietly and imagine the movement.

The nervous system interprets intention as action. As you imagine the movement, you are creating neural connections that will improve your abilities without the strain of excessive effort. Just reading the instructions and "pretending" you are doing the movement actually helps.

Eventually, your movement will become easier. Remember, it took you a lifetime to get to this level of stiffness and fragility. Don't rush the recovery!

Sit on the floor facing the chair with your legs crossed, your right leg in front. Begin to rock to your left, leaning a bit on your left hand. As you rock, let your left thigh touch the ground and let your right knee come up.

Try that rocking movement several times till if feels easy and pleasant. Rest.

Try the same thing to the other side, with your left leg crossed in front. Rest again.

If you decided to stay seated in the chair, just explore rocking from one buttock to another, and notice how the weight shift affects your feet. Feel free to place your hands on the chair seat in front of you.

Return to the first cross-legged position. This time as you rock onto your left buttock, begin to find a way to place the sole of your right foot pressing the floor. Your left hand is also pressing the floor. What is the rest of you doing? Begin to let your whole body turn left. Is there some way you can put your right hand on the floor somewhere by your left leg? Experiment. Where could it support you? What happens if you keep turning? Rest.

Return to sitting with your right leg in front. As you turn further to the left, lower your head a bit as if you wanted to look at your left leg. Support yourself with your hands. You will find yourself kneeling either on your left knee or both knees. Play with that movement a little bit. Take your time, don't force it.

If you have been working in your chair, as you rock, lower your head and press your hands into the chair seat in front of you so that your buttocks come off your seat. If they don't come up, just rock.

Repeat this sequence to the left, then rest.

You could stop right there and you will have learned a lot. You can save the next section for another time, just read the next part and try it later, or go for it. Remember to listen to your comfort level. The following sequence puts the pieces together.

Sit again with your legs crossed, right over left. Rock to your left and come up onto your left knee and right foot. If it's easy with both hands on the floor, slide your right foot up to standing next to your left knee. If this is hard, first place your right hand on the chair seat. Make sure your head is down, looking between your knees. Tuck your left foot as if you were going to stand up. Push your buttocks up in the air, lower your head even more and swivel yourself into the chair like you did in the last chapter. You have now done a complete spiral from the floor to your chair.

If you have been working from sitting in the chair, explore how you can rock and swivel to standing. How much do you need to press the chair seat in front? How long can you keep your head down? Is your breathing relaxed?

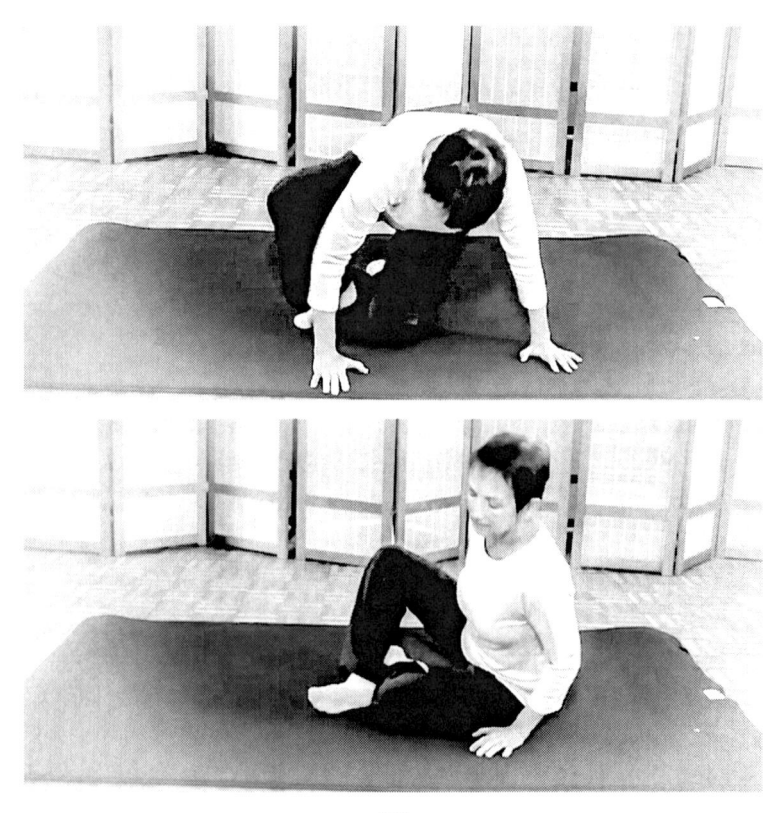

If you wish, you can now swivel from your chair all the way to sitting on the floor and back into your chair. Swivel your knees left. Your right knee lowers to the ground until you are kneeling on your right knee.

In order to sit, shift your weight so that you end up sitting on your right buttock. Lower your head and place your right hand on the floor. Lean to your right till you're sitting on your right buttock. Rock back up to kneeling, then sit again. Take a rest.

If you are sitting on the floor, lie down for a moment. To get back up, just cross your legs, rock, swivel and spiral up to your chair!

Take a few minutes to explore the parts of the movement you enjoyed. Doing any of these movements with attention and care will translate into a more responsive body, which will help in the event of a fall.

After you've finished playing, take another rest. Then get up and take a walk around. Notice if there's something different in the way you walk. Check in with your sense of comfort. Do you feel tired, or like you've exerted yourself? If so, you may have been trying too hard.

Next time, do less, take more breaks, listen to yourself. Our need to push ourselves, to feel that we have to attain some outer idea of perfection often gets in the way of our learning. We tense unnecessarily, cloud our minds with judgment and don't benefit from doing the movement as much.

The Feldenkrais Method is designed to both change the way you move, and the way you think and act. Each time you do one of the lessons in this series, you are carving new neural pathways that will help you keep your balance on your feet and in your life.

Movement is Life: Conclusion

As children, we tumbled, rolled, laid on the grass looking at the stars and then jumped up to chase the dog, leap-frogged over each other falling over sideways, crash-landed after zooming down slides and most of the time somehow managed to get back up. Adulthood in our culture narrows options for movement: driving, sitting at the computer, the TV and meetings put us in the same position. Adults rarely have the urge, let alone the opportunity to swing on a rope, climb a tree or do a somersault unless they are athletes. Somewhere between childhood and the present, life puts constraints on our mobility: injuries, sedentary lifestyle and habits conspire to stiffen and limit us. The earth changes from a welcoming support to a harsh force that doesn't yield to our stiff muscles and fragile bones. The act of falling itself is viewed as a kind of failure and fear of injury increases our potential for damage.

Research shows that the potential for learning is life long. No matter how limited you feel, you can improve. Neuroplasticity, the brain's ability to literally "change itself," can help you re-learn the joy of movement that is your birthright. This book scratches the surface of the human potential for movement, grace and flexibility. I hope it inspires you to include movement into your life, even if only for a few moments, every day. It doesn't matter whether it's dancing, hiking, yoga or just rolling around on the floor.

What does matter is that the movement be varied. Don't just do the same routine every day. Reaching, turning, hopping, bouncing, clambering not only lubricate your joints, these activities also increase your flexibility. Moving can save you hospital bills and painful recovery time, and can provide a more enjoyable approach to every new experience.

In closing, I'd like to propose a radical definition of maturity. Maturity is being unafraid of falling. You are unafraid because you know how to yield to the unknown, you can roll with whatever happens, and you have no need to prove anything by "keeping your head up." A mature individual is one who can hit a bump on the road through life and recover without getting caught in compulsive reactions that make the situation worse. If you fall, whether from grace or off the curb, if you misstep on a mountain path or a career path, you now have many strategies for recovery.

To see the video clips referred to in this book, visit:
goo.gl/B6OsUP

OR SCAN QR CODE

Resources

Products and Information about the Feldenkrais Method

Feldenkrais Guild of North America:
contains a database of practitioners nationwide, articles, info about events and more.
www. feldenkrais.com

The Feldenkrais Store:
is a wonderful online store carrying many audio and video programs covering everything from relaxation to running.
www.thefeldenkraisstore.com

Related Programs

Bones for Life:
This innovative approach to improving bone density and flexibility was developed by Ruthy Alon, a Senior Trainer in the Feldenkrais Method.
www.bonesforlife.com

Change Your Age:
Created by Dr. Frank Wildman, one of Feldenkrais' original US students, the "Change Your Age" program uses Feldenkrais principles to improve fitness and increase power as we age.
www.changeyouragenetwork.com

If you enjoyed this book, and would like to dive deeper into Feldenkrais lessons for this subject, check out Lavinia's Audio Program:

Fall Softly, Recover Quickly
you can order this as a CD set or audio download at
The Feldenkrais Store: www.thefeldenkraisstore.com

And visit www.laviniaplonka.com for more audio downloads

Other titles by Lavinia Plonka

Books:
What Are You Afraid Of? A Body/Mind Guide to Courageous Living
Walking Your Talk: Changing Your Life Through the Magic of Body Language
Playing in the Kitchen
Meditating With My Hair On Fire

Audios:
Unstress Through Movement
The Power of the Pelvis
Have a Comfortable Flight
The Breath Connection

CPSIA information can be obtained
at www.ICGtesting.com
Printed in the USA
LVOW10s1120290617
539691LV00019B/298/P

9 781543 284683